Contents

P349
765'
/HMW AA
(Ree)

Books are to be returned on or before
the last date below

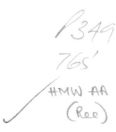

080394862X

Notes on Nursing Theories

SERIES EDITORS

Chris Metzger McQuiston
Doctoral Candidate, Wayne State University

Adele A. Webb
College of Nursing, University of Akron

Notes on Nursing Theories is a series of monographs designed to provide the reader with a concise description of conceptual frameworks and theories in nursing. Each monograph includes a biographical sketch of the theorist, origin of the theory, assumptions, concepts, propositions, examples for application to practice and research, a glossary of terms, and a bibliography of classic works, critiques, and research.

BETTY NEUMAN

The Neuman Systems Model

Karen S. Reed

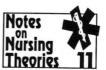
Notes on Nursing Theories 11

SAGE Publications
International Educational and Professional Publisher
Newbury Park   London   New Delhi

For information address:

SAGE Publications, Inc.
2455 Teller Road
Newbury Park, California 91320

SAGE Publications Ltd.
6 Bonhill Street
London EC2A 4PU
United Kingdom

SAGE Publications India Pvt. Ltd.
M-32 Market
Greater Kailash I
New Delhi 110 048 India

Printed in the United States of America

Library of Congress Cataloging-in-Publication Data

Reed, Karen S.
 Betty Neuman: the Neuman systems model / Karen S. Reed.
  p. cm. — (Notes on nursing theories; v. 11)
 Includes bibliographical references.
 ISBN 0-8039-4861-1 (cl). — ISBN 0-8039-4862-X (pb)
 1. Nursing—Philosophy. 2. Neuman, Betty M. 3. Models, Nursing. I. Title. II. Series.
 [DNLM: 1. Neuman, Betty M. 2. Philosophy, Nursing.
 3. Education, Nursing. WY 86 R324b 1993]
 RT84.5.R44 1993
 610.73'01—dc20
 DNLM/DLC   93-26131

   94 95 96 10 9 8 7 6 5 4 3 2

Sage Production Editor: Diane S. Foster

List of Figures

Foreword

Karen Reed's presentation of the Neuman systems model in this easy-to-use, brief format is both timely and pragmatic. Although the intended audience is the undergraduate nursing student, graduate students and faculty alike can avail themselves of this quick and handy resource.

It has been 20 years since Betty Neuman, Ph.D., published the first and primary article on the Neuman systems model in nursing research. Entitled "A Model for Teaching Total Person Approach to Patient Problems," the article reveals Dr. Neuman's creativity and purpose for her work. Nursing students needed a unifying focus in which to place their practice. Twenty years later, nursing students more than ever need to develop a client-centered and holistic context for their learning and their practice.

The Neuman systems model:

- Provides a worldview of nursing that embraces a systems approach
- Maintains the centrality of the client to plans of care
- Clearly establishes nursing as a unique practice that addresses the client system (individual, family, or community) in relationship with the environment

The Neuman systems model systematically describes what occurs in nursing; provides a holistic approach to care; and, when utilized in practice and research, generates new concepts and theories relevant for nursing. To have been a pioneer in the application of the Neuman model to curriculum development and client approach and to have had the privilege of Dr. Neuman's trust and mentorship is to have received the most precious of gifts. Eagerly, I look forward to future developments in the utilization of the Neuman systems model in education, practice, and research that will be undertaken by those undergraduate students who, having availed themselves of this monograph today, become tomorrow's generation of nurse researchers.

I would like to acknowledge the work and wisdom of Karen Reed, Ph.D., for providing the undergraduate student with this primer on the Neuman systems model and Betty Neuman, author and theorist, for her relentless energy and commitment to knowledge development as a "letting go" process.

ROSALIE MIRENDA
Professor, Nursing
Neumann College
Aston, Pennsylvania

Acknowledgments

I am deeply grateful for the support and assistance of Betty Neuman and Rosalie Mirenda during this project. Their encouragement and willingness to help made this assignment the ultimate learning experience.

I also thank Donna Neff for her help in preparing the manuscript.

Biographical Sketch of the Nurse Theorist: Betty Neuman, PhD, RN

Born: 1924, on a farm in southeastern Ohio
Family: Two brothers; husband, Kree; child, Nancy
Educational background: RN, Peoples Hospital, Akron, Ohio,
    1947, as part of the Cadet Nurse Corps; BSN, UCLA, 1957;
    MS in public health-mental health, UCLA, 1966; PhD in
    clinical psychology, Pacific Western University, 1985
Positions: 1967, assumed chairmanship of the program from
    which she had graduated, where she began a program of
    post-master's work for psychiatric nurses in the area of
    community mental health clinical specialty—the first
    such program in the nation; 1978-1979, Curriculum
    Consultant, Ohio University, Athens, Ohio; 1979-1980,
    Continuing Education Director, Ohio University; 1981 to
    present, consultant, lecturer, author
Basic philosophy: Helping each other live

1

Origin of the Theory

In 1970 Dr. Betty Neuman designed a "teaching tool" for use with graduate students. She developed and coordinated a course requested by UCLA graduate nursing students that would provide an overview of course content. Selected faculty presented the overview course, which formed the new programming for clinical specialized teaching in areas such as psychiatric and gerontologic nursing. The purpose of the course was to aid entering graduate students in making appropriate clinical nurse specialization program choices.

A 2-year student evaluation confirmed the value of the "tool" for both course unification and integration of faculty lecture content. It also provided a comprehensive perspective from which to view the entire client situation. Dr. Neuman and a colleague published the diagram entitled "A Total Person Approach to Patient Problems," course evaluation, and results in the spring 1972 issue of *Nursing Research*. To date, the diagram remains unchanged but now is known as the "Neuman systems model." Her early work made explicit to nursing the importance of taking a holistic view of clients through identification of the five client system variables and the importance of their interrelationship with the environment.

Author's Note: The author gratefully acknowledges the extensive use of material provided by Dr. Neuman in the writing of this chapter.

In the first nursing models text, *Conceptual Models for Nursing Practice* (Riehl & Roy, 1974), Riehl classified the original diagram or "tool" for the overview course as a systems model for nursing and titled it the "Betty Neuman health-care systems model," and then added its earlier title, "A Total Person Approach to Patient Problems," when presenting it in their text. Dr. Neuman developed an assessment/intervention tool and other data to clarify further the intent and purpose as well as how to use her work for the Riehl and Roy publication.

Further refinement of the model by Dr. Neuman and others in nursing continues. In 1982 Neuman edited her first book, *The Neuman systems model: Application to Nursing Education and Practice.* In this volume 50 authors joined Dr. Neuman in describing the use of the model in a variety of educational and clinical settings. A more recent edition (Neuman, 1989) expanded on the original work. Plans are in progress for the third edition of the book, which will illustrate the work's increased usage worldwide.

Refinement of model concepts has continued over the past 20 years. Dr. Neuman has incorporated an additional fifth dimension, or variable (spirituality), that was not in the original work. The concept environment was expanded to include the created environment. A nursing process format, an assessment intervention tool, and a prevention-as-intervention process available in the 1974 Riehl and Roy text have been refined and expanded as "tools" for the implementation of the model.

Work continues in the use and clarification of the model in clinical and educational settings. Research focusing on testing of the model has begun. More than 50 countries worldwide are using the model in both educational and practice settings. Thus it is one of the three most widely used nursing models in existence.

Dr. Neuman continues to expand and clarify the model. She sees her present role as both networker and facilitator of the model's use. As such, she spends a large amount of time helping others understand and implement the model in a variety of health settings. During the fall of 1988, as a means to safeguard the integrity and further development of the Neuman systems model, she organized the Neuman systems model Trustees Group, Inc. Dr. Neuman's purpose was to "preserve, protect, and perpetuate the integrity of the Model for the future of nursing" (Neuman, 1989, p. 467).

2

The Neuman systems model: Assumptions and Concepts

Assumptions of the Model

As with many nursing frameworks, the base of Neuman's work is from theoretical foundations outside of nursing. The foundations of Neuman's model are primarily Selye's stress theory, von Bertalanffy's general systems theory, Caplan's levels of prevention, Lewis's field theory, and De Chardin's philosophy of life. These perspectives support the idea that a holistic viewpoint of humans is crucial (Fawcett, 1984). The Neuman model is considered a systems model. In a systems model the main focus is on the interaction of the parts, or subsystems within the system. A systems perspective allows the nurse to view not only the pieces of the puzzle (or subsystems), but also the effect of each piece on all the other pieces. This perspective also illuminates the impact of the system on other systems. This multilevel, multifaceted method of viewing clients is one of the hallmarks of any systems model and, in particular, the Neuman model.

Some basic beliefs about person, health, environment, and nursing are necessary to understand when using the Neuman model. These basic beliefs are called assumptions: They provide the "bottom line" when using a theoretical framework.

5

The following assumptions are found in the Neuman model (Neuman, 1989, pp. 77, 21, 22).

1. Though each individual client or group as a client system is unique, each system is a composite of common known factors or innate characteristics within a normal, given range of response contained within a basic structure.

2. Many known, unknown, and universal environmental stressors exist. Each differs in its potential for disturbing a client's usual stability level, or normal line of defense. The particular interrelationships of client variables—physiological, psychological, sociocultural, developmental, and spiritual—at any point in time can affect the degree to which a client is protected by the flexible line of defense against possible reaction to a single stressor or combination of stressors.

3. Each individual client/client system, over time, has evolved a normal range of response to the environment that is referred to as a normal line of defense, or usual wellness/stability state.

4. When the cushioning, accordionlike effect of the flexible line of defense is no longer capable of protecting the client/client system against an environmental stressor, the stressor breaks through the normal line of defense. The interrelationships of variables—physiological, psychological, sociocultural, developmental, and spiritual—determine the nature and degree of the system reaction or possible reaction to the stressor invasion.

5. The client, whether in a state of wellness or illness, is a dynamic composite of the interrelationships of variables—physiological, psychological, sociocultural, developmental, and spiritual. Wellness is on a continuum of available energy to support the system in its optimal state.

6. Implicit within each client system is a set of internal resistance factors, known as lines of resistance (resources), which function to stabilize and return the client to the usual wellness state (normal line of defense) or possibly to a higher level of stability following an environmental stressor reaction.

7. Primary prevention relates to general knowledge that is applied in client assessment and intervention in identification and reduction or mitigation of risk factors associated with environmental stressors to prevent possible stressor reaction.

8. Secondary prevention relates to symptomatology following a reaction to stressors, appropriate ranking of intervention priorities, and treatment to reduce their noxious effects.

9. Tertiary prevention relates to the adjustive processes taking place as reconstitution begins and maintenance factors move the client back in a circular manner toward primary prevention.
10. The client is in dynamic constant energy exchange with the environment.

Concepts of the Model

Concepts are abstract ideas that describe a collection of thoughts or behaviors that often are hard to pinpoint. Happiness, life, and self-esteem are examples of concepts. Neuman's model concentrates on explaining a person's reaction to stressors in the environment. Six major concepts are used to describe this phenomenon. The major concepts in the model are client, variables, environment, stressors, wellness, and nursing intervention (see Figure 2.1).

Client System

A series of concentric circles surrounding a core, or basic structure, depicts the client system in the Neuman model. Each line of defense or resistance has certain distinct properties, but the main function is to protect the basic structure and help maintain the system in a stable state.

In Neuman's model the term *client* is a synonym for the nursing metaparadigm concept "person." The term *client* indicates a collaborative relationship between caregiver and care receiver and focuses on the wellness perspective of the model. Neuman defines *client* as "an unlimited entity with an active personality system, whose evolution follows principles, symbolism, and systemic organizations . . . It is not always possible to see the potential expansions of this entity and the ramifications of its actions" (Neuman, 1989, p. 11).

In the Neuman model the client can be defined as any system that interacts with the environment. Therefore, the client may be defined as an individual, family, group, or community. The definition used for client depends upon the nurse's population of interest.

Because Neuman believes the client to be open, the relationship of the client to the environment is reciprocal. Therefore, the client both influences and is influenced by the environment. For example, if a

CLIENT	ENVIRONMENT
basic structure	internal
lines of resistance	external
normal line of defense	created
flexible line of defense	

VARIABLES	STRESSORS
physiological	intrapersonal
psychological	interpersonal
developmental	extrapersonal
sociocultural	
spiritual	

NURSING INTERVENTIONS	WELLNESS
primary intervention	entropy
secondary intervention	negentropy
tertiary intervention	
reconstitution	

Figure 2.1. Key Concepts of the Neuman Systems Model
SOURCE: Reprinted by permission of Betty Neuman.

nonsmoker works in an office surrounded by smokers, the individual will be influenced by the environment. He or she may have an increase in respiratory illnesses due to the inhalation of secondary smoke. However, if the nonsmoker circulates a petition to designate smoking and nonsmoking sections within the office environment, he or she is influencing the environment to decrease the stressors.

A circle surrounded by a series of concentric rings graphically represents the client (see Figure 2.2). The rings act as a protective structure for the inner circle, known as the basic structure. The basic structure includes the innate energy resources necessary for the survival of the client. These resources are conceptualized as the survival factors of the species, the genetic features, and strengths and weaknesses of the system parts. For example, if the client is defined as an individual person, then the basic structure would include the mechanisms for maintaining a normal temperature range, the genetic response patterns, and the strength or weakness of body organs (Neuman, 1989).

If a family is considered the client, then the basic structure includes resources for survival of the family unit. This includes the

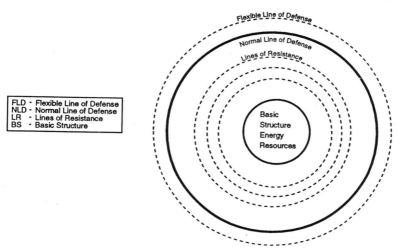

Figure 2.2. The Client System

SOURCE: Adapted from the Neuman systems model diagram, by permission of Betty Neuman.

genetic pool of the individuals within the family, financial resources to maintain the family, and the ethnic or cultural history that provides and maintains the family identity.

The concentric rings around the basic structure (Figure 2.2) form the basis of resource protection for the core of the system. The outer ring, known as the *flexible line of defense* (FLD), forms the outer boundary of the client. This boundary functions to protect the normal line of defense or the usual state of wellness of the client. The flexible line of defense is a buffer for the client and is the first line of defense in response to stressors from the environment. The client uses the flexible line of defense not only to keep the normal state of wellness from being compromised, but also to improve the normal state of wellness. The flexible line of defense is accordionlike in nature, expanding or contracting, depending on the needs of the client. As the flexible line of defense expands it provides more protection; as it contracts, less protection. The ability of the flexible line of defense to function as a buffer relates directly to the type, amount, and strength of stressors within the environment in relationship to the response or reaction of the client. If the number and virility of environmental stressors increase, the buffer system is hard pressed to keep these stressors from impacting the normal functioning of the client. As with a bumper on a car, if the speed of the car increases (increased stressors) and the car comes into contact with a brick wall (increased stressor), the bumper will not be able to protect the car and passengers within the car from damage.

The *normal line of defense* (NLD) is the client's usual state of wellness. It becomes the baseline, or standard of functioning, for the client. The normal line of defense develops over time and is affected by not only internal factors that influence the ability to maintain wellness, but also external factors. External factors influencing the baseline functioning of a client include environmental stressors of a chronic nature (such as pollution, altitude, etc.) to which the client has adapted. Internal factors influencing the baseline functioning include patterns of health behaviors, lifestyle, and cultural influences. If a stressor breaks through the flexible line of defense and comes in contact with the normal line of defense, a reaction will occur within the system. Typically the client will exhibit symptoms of instability or illness, caused by the disruption of the normal stable state.

The *lines of resistance* (LR) are closest to the basic structure and function as a protective mechanism for the basic structure. The main purpose of the lines of resistance is to protect the basic structure's integrity. They become activated following a stressor invasion through the normal line of defense. If the lines of resistance are effective in their protection, the system is able to reconstitute and return to a steady state. When lines of resistance are ineffective, death of the system may occur.

Variables

In earlier writings Neuman (1982) identified only four variables (physiological, sociocultural, psychological, developmental). She since has incorporated the spiritual variable into the model (Neuman, 1989). As she states, "the spiritual variable is viewed as an innate component of the basic structure, whether or not it is ever acknowledged or developed by the client or client system—it influences the system" (Neuman, 1992, personal communication).

According to Neuman, inherent within the client are five different variables. The variables are similar to domains of function within the system. The five variables are: (a) physiological, relating to body structure and function; (b) psychological, dealing with mental processes and relationships; (c) sociocultural, focusing on social and cultural influences; (d) developmental, including life developmental processes; and (e) spiritual, incorporating the belief influences, creative aspects, and essence of life.

The five different variables may be at various levels of development. The variables pertaining to a child are not as developed as those of an adult. There is unlimited potential for interaction among the five variables. A term coined to describe the interaction has been "leaky margins" (personal communication, Beynon, 1991). For example, communication patterns used by the client (a psychological variable) often are influenced by the values of the society in which the client was raised (a sociocultural variable).

Environment

The environment is an important influencing concept of the Neuman model. It is defined as those forces surrounding man, both internal and external (Neuman, 1989). The internal and external environmental stress factors may have a positive or negative influence on the client. In the Neuman model the three environmental typologies identified are *internal, external,* and *created.*

The *internal environment* (intrapersonal) "consists of all forces or interactive influences internal to or contained solely within the boundaries of the client" (Neuman, 1989, p. 31). The internal environment describes the result of relationships among the subsystems of the client. For the individual, this might be the interaction of one body subsystem with another. In a family as client, the interactions of subsystems would be those of the individual family members with one another.

The *external environment* consists of influences of an interpersonal, or extrapersonal, nature. These influences are outside the boundaries of the client. With an individual client the external environment refers to the interaction of the client with another person such as a work colleague or a family member. With a family system as client, the external environment may include extended family or neighbors. Therefore what may be an internal environment to one system may become an external environment to another. The crucial point is in defining the client system as one of interacting parts.

The *created environment*, a newer term to the Neuman systems model, is the client's attempt to create a safe setting for functioning (Neuman, 1990). An environment is created by the client if the client perceives a threat to the basic structure and function of the system. Neuman describes the created environment as largely made up of unconscious mechanisms that come into play as the system interprets the need. The client may use not only internal but also external cues to create a safe haven from which to operate.

An example of creating an environment is the process a person goes through when moving to a new location. The external environment is new and unfamiliar. It is a new city, new state, or new neighborhood. To decrease the feeling of discomfort or threat at the change in environment, one arranges furniture in the new house in a pattern similar to that in the previous home. Patterns of behavior also are kept, such as morning coffee and the newspaper or routines of exercise, all to ease into and feel less vulnerable in a new situation. This rearranging of the environment is not a conscious act to decrease stress. Rather, it is an unconscious attempt to reduce the disparity between the new and unfamiliar and the old and safe. The main goal of a created environment is to maintain system integrity, thereby allowing the system to function in a safe arena. When assessing the existence of a created environment, it is important to consider what environment has been created, how it has been used, and how it will be used by the client to maintain optimal system functioning (Neuman, 1989).

Stressors

Stressors are a part of the environment. Neuman (1989) defines them as "tension producing stimuli with the potential for causing disequilibrium. . . . More than one stressor may be imposed upon the client at any given time" (p. 23). They may be present within or outside the client (see Figure 2.3).

The typology of stressors includes:

1. *Intrapersonal stressors*—internal environmental interaction forces occurring within the boundary of the client, between client subsystems.
2. *Interpersonal stressors*—external environmental interaction forces occurring outside the boundary of the client but at proximal range.

Stressors
- Identified
- Classified as to knows or possibilities, i.e.
  - Loss
  - Pain
  - Sensory deprivation
  - Cultural change

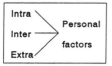

Stressors
- More than one stressor could occur simultaneously
- Same stressors could vary as to impact or reaction
- Normal defense line varies with age and development

Figure 2.3. Stressors Within the Environment

SOURCE: Adapted from the Neuman systems model diagram, by permission of Betty Neuman.

3. *Extrapersonal stressors*—external environmental interaction forces occurring outside the boundary of the client at distal range.

The stressor's effect on the client is related to two factors: (a) the strength of the stressor and (b) the number of stressors impinging on the client at any given time. However, the stressor's effect also is related to the client's ability to protect against the stressor or change its effect on the system. Therefore, each client may have a different reaction to similar environmental stressors.

For example, an individual who makes a decision to return to school for an advanced degree may decide to continue working full time. However, few students are able to manage the additional stress if they are enrolled full time in school while working full time. The additional stress of class attendance, homework, and faculty expectations to the normal stress load typically decreases sleep time, disrupts patterns of eating and exercise, and reduces leisure time. Such activities help maintain the flexible line of defense. Therefore the student has weakened the flexible line of defense and may find herself more susceptible to infections and disease, thus becoming ill when she can least afford to.

Wellness

In the Neuman model, health status is reflected by the level of client *wellness*. Health and wellness are considered to be the same (Neuman, 1989). When system needs are fully met, a state of optimal wellness exists and the client is healthy. Conversely, unmet needs reduce the wellness state. Wellness is a condition where all subsystems are in balance and harmony with the whole of the client. Varying degrees of health exist, depending on the balance between met and unmet needs of the client. Thus health is on a continuum from wellness to illness. The wellness of the client is based upon the actual or potential effect that environmental stressors have on the energy level of the system. For example, it requires less energy output to maintain a high degree of wellness for a client if the environment does not include air and water pollution.

When more energy is produced than used, the client is moving toward *negentropy,* or a wellness state. When the system produces less energy than is required, movement of the client is toward *entropy,* or illness (Neuman, 1989). The greater the entropy state, the greater the imbalance between the needs of the system and the energy available. Energy conservation is critical to the goal of system stability.

Nursing Interventions

Nursing's goal is to keep the client stable. In systems terms, the maintenance of stability requires that interventions are directed toward counteracting movement toward entropy, or illness. Neuman (1989) describes nursing interventions by using the term *prevention.* The three types of prevention are (a) *primary,* (b) *secondary,* and (c) *tertiary.* The three levels of prevention are used to attain, maintain, and retain wellness by assisting system stability (see Figure 2.4).

Primary prevention is intervention aimed at protecting the normal line of defense by (a) increasing the flexible line of defense's ability to withstand environmental stressors and (b) decreasing risk factors. Nurses use *secondary prevention* interventions when the normal line of defense is disrupted, resulting in client symptoms. Secondary

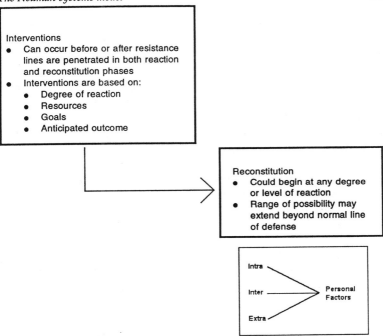

Figure 2.4. Levels of Prevention, Reconstitution

SOURCE: Adapted from the Neuman systems model diagram, by permission of Betty Neuman.

prevention is aimed at strengthening the system's lines of resistance and thus protecting the basic structure (see Figure 2.4). *Tertiary prevention* focuses on helping the client regain or return to a wellness state following treatment. The term *reconstitution* describes the process of returning to a wellness state. "Reconstitution may be viewed as feedback from the input and output of secondary intervention. The goal is to maintain an optimal wellness level by supporting existing strengths and conserving client energy" (Neuman, 1989, p. 37).

The Neuman model provides a framework from which to view the person as a system based on systems theory. The concepts— client system, variables, environment, stressors, wellness, and nursing interventions—are derived from a variety of systems-, stress-, and mental health-related theories. The Neuman model is built on the assumption that the interaction of environment and client has both direct and indirect effects on the client's ability to maintain a state of wellness. The goal of nursing is to provide assistance for the client to best attain and maintain system stability as an optimal condition of wellness. When it becomes impossible for the client to conserve energy, the client is assisted in a peaceful and meaningful death.

In conclusion, the Neuman systems model is comprised of six major concepts that explain and examine the interaction of persons with the environment. The Neuman model provides a framework for describing the process that occurs as clients maintain, attain, or retain health during encounters with stressors. It is a multilevel, multidimensional systems model that allows for describing very complex situations (see Figúre 2.5).

The Neuman Nursing Process

The nursing process as identified by Neuman includes all the common steps of the nursing process: assessment, planning, intervention, and evaluation. However, it was "designed specifically for nursing implementation of the Neuman systems model" (Neuman, 1989, p. 40) and contains three steps: nursing diagnosis, nursing goals, and nursing outcomes. The Neuman nursing process is used in conjunction with the "prevention-as-intervention" format, which is described later.

A nursing diagnosis is derived following assessment of the impact of stressors or potential stressors on the client system and the relative strength of the client system. The assessment process provides the evidence for a diagnostic statement that accurately describes the client's condition. Once the diagnosis is developed, it becomes the basis for nursing goals and outcomes. Nursing goals are developed to assist the client toward retaining a state of wellness. Nursing outcomes are determined by using primary, secondary, or tertiary interventions as necessary and evaluating the outcome goals once intervention has taken place.

A unique aspect of the Neuman nursing process is the emphasis on client input. In the first step the nurse verifies her or his perceptions with the client in terms of the meaning of the stressor and the strengths and weaknesses of the system. Client input also is important in terms of the nursing goals and evaluating outcome. Client

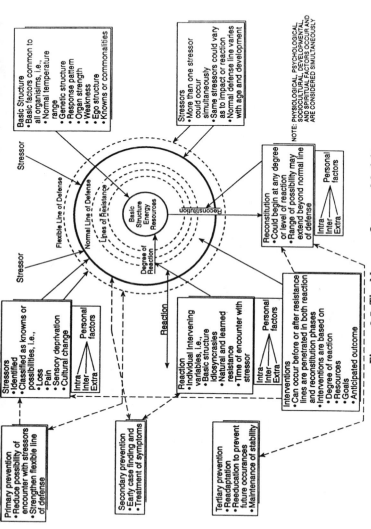

Figure 2.5. The Neuman Systems Model

NOTE: Spiritual variable added.

SOURCE: Reprinted by permission of Betty Neuman.

17

negotiation is viewed as necessary in formulating the nursing intervention goals. Intervention outcomes also are verified with the client.

Utilizing the Neuman Nursing Process With an Individual Client System

The following is an example of the use of the Neuman nursing process with an individual.

Case Example

Mr. L is a 49-year-old divorced male with two children. He has come to the clinic to seek help for depression following the breakup of a long-term relationship. For the past 3 weeks he has had difficulty sleeping and concentrating. He obsessively thinks about the woman he was involved with. Mr. L finds himself crying and feeling as if his world has ended. He denies wanting to harm himself or others.

Mr. L has been divorced for 15 years. His marriage was a stormy one that lasted 12 years. Since that time he has been involved in a series of relationships. Only two were serious enough to think of marriage, including this most recent one. The last relationship was of 1½ years' duration.

Mr. L has a history of seven hospitalizations in his life. Three of these hospitalizations were for acute pancreatitis, and one was for treatment of acute gastritis. Mr. L acknowledges that he used to drink alcohol on a regular basis, but for the past 8 months has maintained sobriety. He smokes approximately two packs of cigarettes per day. He appears slightly overweight and looks older than his stated age. His blood pressure is elevated at 180/90. There is a history of cardiac disease on his maternal side; his paternal side is negative for major physical illness, but is positive for unipolar and bipolar depression. He eats most of his meals at fast-food restaurants and rarely cooks at home. He does little physical activity outside of his job, which is fairly sedentary.

Mr. L has had custody of his children since they were ages 12 and 10. Both children have graduated from high school in the past 3 years and are gainfully employed. Mr. L himself did not finish high school, but obtained a GED while in the army. He has been employed at the same factory since being discharged from the army.

Mr. L's family lives in the area. He is not particularly close to any of them and sees them infrequently. His relationship with his children is at present tenuous. His younger child, a son, is contemplating moving back home so he can go to school. Since Mr. L's last bout with alcohol, his daughter has refused to speak with him.

Mr. L does not have any hobbies or leisure activities that he pursues on a regular basis. He admits to being "crazy about cars" and has in the past bought several classic cars in order to restore them. However, he tends to lose interest in the middle of the project and often must pay others to complete the restorations. He spends most of his time working at the factory and seeing his friends in the bar. He acknowledges that this has been difficult for him lately, since he is trying to maintain sobriety.

When asked to clarify why he has sought help, he states that he is tired of choosing the wrong kind of woman to have a relationship with and wants to learn how to make better choices. He cannot understand why his last girlfriend decided she needed to see other people and why their relationship wasn't enough to satisfy her.

The Neuman Nursing Process Applied

  I. Nursing Diagnosis
    A. Database
      1. Actual and potential stressors
        a. Actual: Mr. L has experienced the breakup of a long-term relationship, he recently quit drinking, and his relationship with his daughter is strained.
        b. Potential: Mr. L's adult child (son) is planning to move back into his home; there is a possibility of a relapse of alcoholic behavior. Mr. L has a potential for suicidal behavior.
      2. Structure assessment
        a. Basic structure (strengths and weaknesses): Mr. L is moderately obese and has a family history of alcoholism, cardiac disease, and depression. He has a history of alcohol use. Mr. L is financially stable at the present time. He has a history of difficulty maintaining close relationships with females.

  b. Lines of defense, resistance (strengths and weaknesses): Mr. L is a well-groomed, articulate 49-year-old male. He completed a GED while in the army. Mr. L has been gainfully employed at the same institution for 23 years. He has maintained sobriety for 8 months. There is no suicidal ideation present. Mr. L recognizes the need for help. He has experienced difficulty sleeping through the night and difficulty concentrating for the past 6 weeks. Mr. L has little insight into problems regarding romantic female relationships. He feels that others are responsible for most of his problems. Mr. L does no physical exercise on a regular basis. He eats out at restaurants and his diet is high in fat and sodium. Mr. L works the swing shift at the local factory, which limits his ability to establish a routine regarding sleep habits. Mr. L's leisure time is spent in bars. Since sobriety, he continues to go to the bars, but drinks nonalcoholic beer. His relationship with his daughter is poor; his relationship with his son is good. Male friendships are limited to casual acquaintances. Mr. L has little interaction with other family members.

B. Variances From Wellness

  1. Synthesis of theory: The client has a weakened flexible line of defense as evidenced by lack of healthy routines established to help him cope with stressors. His past coping mechanisms have focused on the use of alcohol. Few psychological resources are utilized at present, as evidenced by the lack of social support and an unwillingness to look at the interpersonal dynamics of the situation. Mr. L prefers to blame others for his problems. There is a need for an external support system to stabilize the client system and begin reconstitution. Mr. L's structure is intact, but there are inherent weaknesses related to a familial history of alcoholism, cardiac illness, and depression.

  2. Hypothetical interventions: Provide psychoeducational readings on dependent behaviors, alcoholism, and medications. Monitor effects of antidepressant medications. Work with client to modify physical activity routines and dietary habits. Encourage Mr. L to develop hobbies, and to increase interaction with others. Family counseling with son and daughter is recommended.

II. Nursing Goals

   A. Mr. L is willing to read materials on dependency and on medications. He refuses to discuss alcohol intake and states it is not a problem: "I've been sober for 8 months. I can control my drinking."

   B. Mr. L recognizes the need for changes in dietary habits and exercise routines. He sets a goal of walking twice a week for 45 minutes.

   C. Mr. L refuses to enter into family counseling with son and daughter. He states he doesn't need to be lectured by his daughter. He does agree to meet with the counselor after discharge to discuss his interpersonal problems with females.

III. Nursing Outcomes

   A. Readings given to Mr. L on dependent personalities and on antidepressant medication.

   B. Dietary guidelines given and discussed. A dietary plan for home is worked out.

   C. Information is given to the son and daughter regarding support groups for Adult Children of Alcoholics.

Intervention Format of the Neuman Model: Prevention as Intervention

One of the areas of the Neuman systems model that has received considerable attention and is in wide use is the prevention-as-intervention format of the model. Both Neuman (1989) and Fawcett (1989) believe the "prevention-as-intervention format" is the beginning of an important theory to be derived from the Neuman model. However, concepts as yet have not been operationally defined or linked with specific propositions.

Neuman describes the prevention-as-intervention format as a typology. This means it is a way to view the links between environmental stressors; the reaction of the client to stressors; and the role of nursing in helping clients to retain, attain, or maintain wellness. The three levels described in the prevention-as-intervention format are primary, secondary, and tertiary.

In primary prevention the goal is the retention of wellness. Wellness is retained by strengthening the flexible line of defense and reducing risk factors. Primary prevention interventions concentrate on decreasing the amount of stress in the environment or on increasing the client's ability to withstand stress. Increasing the ability to withstand stress, in Neuman model terms, is known as strengthening the flexible line of defense. Thus, the goal of primary prevention intervention is to protect the client system's normal line of defense, or functioning at an optimal level.

Intervention may occur any time an actual or potential stressor is identified. Potential stressors are situations that have the potential for disrupting the client system. In potential stressful situations the client system has not yet reacted to the stressor. For example, if the client system is identified as an expectant family, a potential stressor for the system would be the introduction of a new member into the system. Primary prevention activities for the parents might include attendance at prenatal classes to prepare for childbirth. In Neuman terms this would be considered a measure to strengthen the family unit's flexible line of defense. Primary prevention also would include helping the parents look at ways to reduce the amount of stress in their environment by changing work schedules and increasing support systems.

Secondary prevention is used any time a reaction to a stressor occurs and the normal state of wellness is disrupted, resulting in overt symptoms being identified. In secondary prevention the goal is to protect the client's basic functioning and facilitate a return to wellness. In Neuman terms this means that because stressors have penetrated the normal line of defense, the internal lines of resistance must be strengthened to protect the basic structure. This strengthening is done by providing appropriate treatment, utilizing client resources, and helping the client conserve energy to deal with the stressor effects.

To use the previous illustration, suppose the birth of the child was premature. Such an event would increase the strength of the original stressor, the addition of a family member. As such, the stressor has broken through the normal line of defense (state of wellness) for the family unit. This breakthrough is evidenced by the infant's hospitalization and the overt stress symptoms in the family. Symptoms seen within the family might include tension between parents, other siblings seeking increased attention from parents, financial strain on the family unit, physical exhaustion, and changes in work arrangements to be with the infant. Secondary prevention interventions would focus on the symptoms of system distress. These interventions would include actions such as providing opportunities for the family to witness the caregiving of the infant, teaching the parents about a premature infant, and helping the family mobilize adequate or needed support from outside resources.

Tertiary prevention is used to maintain wellness after treatment by supporting existing strengths and conserving client system energy. Tertiary prevention is closely linked to reconstitution. Reconstitution is defined as "the return and maintenance of system stability, following treatment of stressor reaction" (Neuman, 1989, p. 50). Because of stressor invasion the client system may or may not return to the previous level of wellness that was available before the stressor impact. Interventions at the tertiary level focus on helping the client system attain or maintain the best possible level of wellness following treatment and help the client conserve as much energy as possible.

Using the previous example, tertiary prevention would focus on helping the family incorporate a premature infant into the home following discharge from the hospital. This incorporation includes providing education and comfort to the family as well as monitoring the infant's physical and developmental progress. It also includes continuing to support parents as needed and determined by the parents in concert with the nurse.

3

Application to Practice and Research

In the past 20 years the use of the Neuman systems model to guide practice and research has grown exponentially. In the beginning the model was primarily used in academia, fulfilling Neuman's original idea that the model should be used as a teaching aid (Neuman, 1989). Initially the model was used as a teaching method. Subsequently the model was used to organize the entire nursing curricula. The nursing program at Neumann College in Aston, Pennsylvania, was the first college to do so, in the early 1970s. Since that time numerous colleges and universities around the nation and the world have based both baccalaureate and graduate nursing programs on the model.

With students becoming cognizant and comfortable with the model during their educational experience, the next logical step was an increase in the application of the model in practice and research. In both editions of Neuman's book (1982, 1989), the vast majority of the material presented focuses on the application of the model in practice and research. Examples of application are not limited to these two volumes. A listing of material found in the literature that utilizes the Neuman systems model is included in the bibliography. Several of the sources included in the bibliography are discussed here in further detail as examples of how the Neuman model has been utilized in practice and research.

Practice

Individual Client Systems

The Neuman systems model has been utilized to describe individuals, families, and communities as client systems. With the individual as client system, the Neuman model has been used to support assessment and intervention models for a variety of age groups and clinical situations. The model has been used to develop a method of assessing nutritional status in both newborns (Torkington, 1988) and adult populations (Gavan, Hastings-Tolsma, & Troyan, 1988). Moore and Munro (1990) used the model to describe a method of assessing the mental health needs of older adults, and Herrick, Goodykoontz, Herrick, and Kackett (1991) developed a continuum of care for disturbed children: "The continuum provides a guide for nurses and other health care providers to achieve high quality care as economically as possible" (p. 41).

The Neuman model has been used in working with clients with multiple sclerosis (MS). Knight (1990) reports that the model is especially effective in describing the MS patient because the open system approach to viewing clients allows for the complex and often unpredictable situations found in MS clients. Brown (1988) used the model to examine risk-factor reduction in myocardial infarction patients, as well as to develop a plan of care.

Family Client Systems

Several authors have described the use of the Neuman model in assessment and planning of care for families in a variety of situations. Beckingham and Baumann (1990) presented an assessment and decision-making model for use with elderly families. Included is a schematic model of assessment that delineates the steps necessary for assessing elderly clients. With the same population, Delunas (1990) describes the process of assessing families who are at high risk for elder abuse. Using the model, an assessment system is iterated that focuses on intra-, inter-, and extra family stressors, giving nurses a means to assess the family as to their ability to care for an elder in the home without risk of abuse.

On the other end of the age spectrum, Wallingford (1989) describes the ability of the Neuman model to provide a framework for caring for families with a neurologically impaired child, including preparation for death. The stress of an impaired member, especially a child, can be devastating to a family. The article goes step by step to describe the impact of the chronic illness on the family system and specifies ways in which the nurse can help the family reconstitute.

The family and its interaction with the community also has been investigated. Authors such as Buchanan (1987) and Story and Ross (1986) describe the development of family assessment in community health nursing. One project that has been implemented is the system at the Middlesex-London Health Unit in London, Ontario. This health unit has implemented a family-based service model for the entire nursing division of the public health department (Drew, Craig, & Beynon, 1989).

Research

Use of the Neuman model as a conceptual framework for research has increased remarkably in the past 10 years. As examples, four studies are used here to illustrate the state of research with the Neuman model.

The Neuman model was used as a basis for an interview guide in a research study that examined the needs of cancer patients and their caregivers (Blank, Clark, Longman, & Atwood, 1989). The interview guides were developed to assess patient and caregiver stressors. Stressors were categorized as intra-, inter-, and extrapersonal. The authors state, "The Neuman Framework is most appropriate for the purpose of addressing the home-care needs of cancer patients and their caregivers" (Blank et al., 1989, p. 81).

Leja (1989) investigated the effectiveness of guided imagery on depressed elderly clients following surgery using a quasi-experimental, nonequivalent control group design. The hypotheses for the study were that (a) older adults would have significantly lower depression scored 1 week following guided imagery teaching and (b) subjects who received guided imagery teaching would have significantly lower depression scores than subjects who received regular discharge teaching. Patients were asked to complete the Beck Depression Inventory prior to discharge. Following completion of the inventory, patients in the experimental group received guided imagery teaching; those in the control group received standard discharge teaching. Depression inventories were then mailed to the participants following discharge, with instructions to complete and return the material to the researcher.

Results of the study showed that patients who received guided imagery teaching did have lower scores of depression following discharge. This supported the first hypothesis. However, there was no difference between the experimental and control groups in postdischarge depression scores. Both groups were less depressed following discharge, no matter what type of intervention was used. Therefore, the author was not able to conclude that guided imagery was more effective than regular discharge teaching. The lack of support for the hypothesis may have been due to the small sample size ($n = 10$). However, the author identified discharge following surgical hospitalization as an additional stressor and the use of guided imagery as a primary prevention measure.

Ali and Khalil (1989) used the Neuman model to provide the theoretical rationale for studying the effect of psychoeducational preparation on patients' anxiety levels prior to cancer surgery. They hypothesized that the stress of a cancer diagnosis and the anticipation of surgery would increase the anxiety level of patients, thus weakening the flexible line of defense for the patients. The treatment, psychoeducational preparation, was to "raise the patients' line of defense and reduce their anxiety post operatively and before discharge" (Ali & Khalil, 1989, p. 238). The findings of the study supported their hypotheses and interventions.

Areas of congruence between personal and contextual factors and the assumptions of the Neuman model were explored by Hinds (1990). Quality-of-life issues were examined with a sample of lung cancer patients ($n = 87$). The seven factors studied accounted for 30% of the explained variance in reports of quality of life among the patients. Hinds described the fit of Neuman's assumptions with the client population. Lung cancer patients were described as systems whose "basic client structure is under attack and client survival is threatened" (Hinds, 1990, p. 460).

Evidence of testing of the Neuman model can be found in the literature. Hoch (1987) compared the Roy's adaptation model and Neuman's model. She found no difference in the two approaches to patient care, but did find a significant difference when comparing the groups who had nursing-theory-based care to those who did not. Quayhagen and Roth (1989) analyzed the fit of the Neuman model with available family assessment measurements. They identified 20 different scales, indexes, and inventories needed to measure the conceptual domains in the Neuman framework. Reed (in press) describes the process in developing a family assessment model to test placement of family concepts within the Neuman model.

In summary, the Neuman model is well represented in the nursing literature. The model is utilized in a wide variety of clinical settings with many different client populations. It has proven to be a most popular mechanism for structuring nursing care. Research supporting the model's concepts is at a beginning level of sophistication. Much work is needed in the area of concept development and measurement of constructs.

Glossary

Central core

The basic structure of survival factors "common to the species, such as variables contained within, innate or genetic factors, and strength and weakness of the system parts" (Neuman, 1989, p. 172).

Client/client system

An open system in interaction with the environment, comprised of variables (physiological, psychological, sociocultural, developmental, and spiritual) that form the whole of the client. The client as a system is composed of a core or basic structure of survival factors and surrounding protective concentric rings. The client system may be an individual, group, family, or community (Neuman, 1989).

Created environment

Unconsciously developed by the client as a "symbolic expression of system wholeness." It is intrapersonal, interpersonal, and extrapersonal in nature. The created environment supersedes and encompasses both internal and external environments (Neuman, 1989, p. 70).

Client system stability

The best possible health state at any given point, where all variables are in balance or harmony with the whole of the client or client system.

29

Developmental variable
Developmental processes of client system.

Environment
All internal and external factors or influences surrounding the identified client or client system. The relationship between the client or client system and the environment is reciprocal. "Input, output and feedback between the client and environment is of a circular nature [such that] the client may influence or be influenced by environmental forces" (Neuman, 1989, p. 70).

External environment
All forces or interaction influences external to or existing outside the defined client or client system.

Extrapersonal factor
Forces occurring outside the client system.

Family
Primary system responsible for the transmission of social values, psychological growth, and spiritual strength of its members who reside within the system. These functions are transmitted through bonds developed by the interrelatedness and communication of individual members (Reed, 1989, p. 385).

Flexible line of defense
A "dynamic state of wellness; system's current, immediate state which is particularly susceptible to situational circumstances; e.g., amount of sleep, hormone level" (Neuman, 1982, p. 137). The flexible line of defense is the boundary between the client system and the environment.

Goal of nursing
To: "facilitate for the client optimal wellness through either retention, attainment or maintenance of client system stability. . . . To assist the client in creating and shaping reality in a desired direction, related to retention, attainment and/or maintenance of optimal system wellness through purposeful interventions . . . directed at mitigation or reduction of stress factors and adverse conditions which affect or could affect optimal client functioning, at any given point of time." (Neuman, 1989, p. 72)

Health
Health "is reflected in the level of wellness. When system needs are met, a state of optimal wellness exists; conversely, unmet needs reduce the wellness state" (Neuman, 1989, p. 71).

Internal environment
All forces or interactive influences internal to or contained solely within the boundaries of the defined client or client system (Neuman, 1989).

Interpersonal factor
A force occurring among two or more client systems.

Intrapersonal factor
A force occurring within the individual.

Lines of resistance
Internal resistant forces that act to decrease the degree of reaction to stressors. They act as resources to help the client return to a stable health condition (personal communication, Neuman, 1992).

Normal line of defense
Adaptational state to stressors over time that is considered "normal" for the individual (Neuman, 1989).

Nursing diagnosis
"Acquisition of an appropriate date base that identifies, assesses, classifies, and evaluates the dynamic interactions among the physiological, psychological, sociocultural, developmental, and spiritual variables comprising the client system. This step of the nursing process takes into account the perceptions of both the client and the caregiver" (Fawcett, 1989, p. 177).

Nursing outcomes
Determined by nursing interventions using one or more of the three prevention modes (Neuman, 1989). Outcomes are the desired results of nursing interventions and are stated behaviorally in terms of the patient. They are derived from the nursing diagnoses and correlate with them. They are classified as short term and long term; they also may be classified as immediate, intermediate, and future. Outcomes will change as the patient/client's status and priorities change. The actual outcomes of the prescribed nursing interventions are evalu-

ated in terms of their relation to the stated outcomes (Neuman, 1989).

Neuman Nursing Process

Designed to implement and facilitate the use of the Neuman systems model for nursing. The nursing process has been systemized into three categories: nursing diagnosis, nursing goals, and nursing outcomes.

Physiologic variable

Bodily structure and function of the client system.

Prevention as intervention

Modes for facilitating integrative processes necessary to retain/ attain/maintain stability and integrity of the client or client system. Intervention modes are used within the structure of each of the preventions: primary, secondary, and tertiary (Neuman, 1989).

Primary prevention

Relates to general knowledge that is applied to individual patient assessment in an attempt to identify and allay the possible risk factors associated with environmental stressors. Decreases the possibility of encounter with stressors and strengthens the flexible line of defense in the system to protect the integrity of the normal line of defense.

Psychological variable

Mental processes and relationships of the client system.

Reconstitution

"Represents the return and maintenance of system stability, following treatment of stressor reaction, which may result in a higher or lower level of wellness than previously" (Neuman, 1989, p. 50).

Sociocultural variable

Social and cultural functions of the client system.

Spiritual variable

"Aspects of spirituality. A continuum from complete unawareness or denial to a consciously developed high level of spiritual understanding" (Neuman, 1989).

Stressor

"Any environmental stimulus, problem, or condition capable of causing instability of the system by penetration of the normal line of defense; this may be intra-, inter-, or extrapersonal in nature" (Neuman, 1982, p. 137).

Secondary prevention

Relates to symptomatology, appropriate ranking of intervention priorities, and treatment protocol. Treats system response following stressor penetration of normal line of defense.

Tertiary prevention

Relates to the adaptive process as reconstitution begins, and ultimately moves back in a circular manner toward primary prevention. Assists in repatterning for restoration of the functions that have been altered as a consequence of the response to stressor penetration of the normal line of defense.

Variances from wellness

Determined by comparing the normal health state with what is taking place at a given time period (Neuman, 1989).

References

Ali, N. S., & Khalil, H. Z. (1989). Effect of psychoeducational intervention on anxiety among Egyptian bladder cancer patients. *Cancer Nursing, 12,* 236-242.

Beckingham, A. C., & Baumann, A. (1990). The aging family in crisis: Assessment and decision-making models. *Journal of Advanced Nursing, 15,* 782-787.

Blank, J. J., Clark, L., Longman, A. J., & Atwood, J. R. (1989). Perceived home care needs of cancer patients and their caregivers. *Cancer Nursing, 12,* 78-84.

Brown, M. W. (1988). Neuman's systems model in risk factor reduction. *Cardiovascular Nursing, 24*(6), 43.

Buchanan, B. F. (1987). Human-environment interaction: A modification of the Neuman systems model for aggregates, families, and the community. *Public Health Nursing, 4,* 52-64.

Delunas, L. R. (1990). Prevention of elder abuse: Betty Neuman health care systems approach. *Clinical Nurse Specialist, 4,* 54-58.

Drew, L. L., Craig, D. M., & Beynon, C. E. (1989). The Neuman systems model for community health administration and practice: Provinces of Manitoba and Ontario, Canada. In B. Neuman (Ed.), *The Neuman systems model* (2nd ed.) (pp. 315-342). Norwalk, CT: Appleton & Lange.

Fawcett, J. (1984). *Analysis and evaluation of conceptual models of nursing.* Philadelphia: F. A. Davis.

Fawcett, J. (1989). *Analysis and evaluation of conceptual models of nursing* (2nd ed.). Philadelphia: F. A. Davis.

Gavan, C. A. S., Hastings-Tolsma, M. T., & Tryan, P. J. (1988). Explication of Neuman's model: A holistic systems approach to nutrition for health promotion in the life process. *Holistic Nursing Practice, 3*(1), 26-38.

Herrick, C. A., Goodykoontz, L., Herrick, R. H., & Kacket, B. (1991). Planning a continuum of care in child psychiatric nursing: A collaborative effort. *Journal of Child and Adolescent Psychiatric and Mental Health Nursing, 4,* 41-48.

Hinds, C. (1990). Personal and contextual factors predicting patients' reported quality of life: Exploring congruency with Betty Neuman's assumptions. *Journal of Advanced Nursing, 15,* 456-462.

Hoch, C. C. (1987). Assessing delivery of nursing care . . . Roy adaptation model and the Neuman health care systems model . . . increasing life satisfaction in retired individuals. *Journal of Gerontological Nursing, 13*(1), 10-17.

Knight, J. B. (1990). The Betty Neuman systems model applied to practice: A client with multiple sclerosis. *Journal of Advanced Nursing, 15,* 447-455.

Leja, A. M. (1989). Using guided imagery to combat postsurgical depression. *Journal of Gerontological Nursing, 15*(4), 6-11.

Moore, S. L., & Munro, M. F. (1990). The Neuman systems model applied to mental health nursing of older adults. *Journal of Advanced Nursing, 15,* 293-299.

Neuman, B. (1982). *The Neuman systems model: Application to nursing education and practice.* New York: Appleton-Century-Crofts.

Neuman, B. (1989). *The Neuman systems model* (2nd ed.). Norwalk, CT: Appleton & Lange.

Neuman, B. M. (1990). Health as a continuum based on the Neuman systems model. *Nursing Science Quarterly, 3,* 129-135.

Quayhagen, M. P., & Roth, P. A. (1989). From models to measures in assessment of mature families. *Journal of Professional Nursing, 5,* 144-151.

Reed, K. (1993). Adapting the Neuman systems model for family nursing. *Nursing Science Quarterly, 6*(2), 93-97.

Reed, K. S. (1989). Family theory related to the Neuman systems model. In B. Neuman (Ed.), *The Neuman systems model* (2nd ed.) (pp. 385-395). Norwalk, CT: Appleton & Lange.

Riehl, J. P., & Roy, C. (1974). *Conceptual models for nursing practice.* New York: Appleton-Century-Crofts.

Story, E. L., & Ross, M. M. (1986). Family centered community health nursing and the Betty Neuman systems model. *Nursing Papers, Perspectives in Nursing, 18,* 77-88.

Torkington, S. (1988). Nourishing the infant. *Senior Nurse, 8*(2), 24-25.

Wallingford, P. (1989). The neurologically impaired and dying child: Applying the Neuman systems model. *Issues in Comprehensive Pediatric Nursing, 12,* 139-157.

Bibliography

References Related to Neuman's Work

Aggleton, P., & Chalmers, H. (1989). Neuman's systems model. *Nursing Times, 85*(51), 27-29.

Ali, N. S., & Khalil, H. Z. (1989). Effect of psychoeducational intervention on anxiety among Egyptian bladder cancer patients. *Cancer Nursing, 12,* 236-242.

Baerg, K. L. (1991). Using Neuman's model to analyze a clinical situation. *Rehabilitation Nursing, 16,* 38-39.

Barrett, M. (1991). A thesis is born. *Image: Journal of Nursing Scholarship, 23,* 261-262.

Bass, L. S. (1991). What do parents need when their infant is a patient in the NICU? *Journal of Neonatal Nursing, 10*(1), 25-38.

Beckingham, A. C., & Baumann, A. (1990). The aging family in crisis: Assessment and decision-making models. *Journal of Advanced Nursing, 15,* 782-787.

Berkey, K. M., & Hanson, S. M. H. (1991). *Family assessment and intervention.* St. Louis, MO: C. V. Mosby.

Beyea, S., & Matzo, M. (1989). Assessing elders using the functional health pattern assessment model. *Nurse Educator, 14*(5), 32-37.

Biley, F. (1990). The Neuman model: An analysis. *Nursing* (London), *4*(4), 25-28.

Biley, F. C. (1989). Stress in high dependency units. *Intensive Care Nursing, 5,* 134-141.

Blank, J. J., Clark, L., Longman, A. J., & Atwood, J. R. (1989). Perceived home care needs of cancer patients and their caregivers. *Cancer Nursing, 12,* 78-84.

Bonner, M., Sr. (Ed.). (1988). *Proceedings of the First International Nursing Symposium, Neuman systems model.* Aston, PA: Neumann College Nursing Program.

Bourbonnais, F. F., & Ross, M. M. (1985). The Neuman systems model in nursing education, course development and implementation. *Journal of Advanced Nursing, 10*, 117-123.

Bowdler, J. E., & Barrell, L. M. (1987). Health needs of homeless persons. *Public Health Nursing, 4*, 135-140.

Breckenridge, D. M., Cupit, M. C., & Raimond, J. N. (1982). Systematic nursing assessment tool for the CAPD client. *Nephrology Nurse, 24*, 26-27, 30-31.

Brown, M. W. (1988). Neuman's systems model in risk factor reduction. *Cardiovascular Nursing, 24*(6), 43.

Buchanan, B. F. (1987). Human-environment interaction: A modification of the Neuman systems model for aggregates, families, and the community. *Public Health Nursing, 4*, 52-64.

Burke, S. O., & Maloney, R. (1986). The women's value orientation questionnaire: An instrument revision study. *Nursing Papers, 18*(1), 32-44.

Burritt, J. E. (1988). The effects of perceived social support on the relationship between job stress and job satisfaction and job performance among registered nurses employed in acute care facilities. *Dissertation Abstracts International, 49*, 2123B.

Campbell, V. (1989). The Betty Neuman health care systems model: An analysis. In J. P. Riehl-Sisca (Ed.), *Conceptual models for nursing* (3rd ed.) (pp. 63-72). Norwalk, CT: Appleton & Lange.

Cantin, B., & Mitchell, M. (1989). Nurses' smoking behavior. *The Canadian Nurse, 85*(1), 20-21.

Capers, C. F. (1986). Some basic facts about models, nursing conceptualizations, and nursing theories. *Journal of Continuing Education in Nursing, 17*, 149-154.

Carroll, T. L. (1989). Role deprivation in baccalaureate nursing students pre and post curriculum revision. *Journal of Nursing Education, 28*, 134-139.

Clark, C. C., Cross, J. R., Deane, D. M., & Lowry, L. W. (1991). Spirituality: Integral to quality care. *Holistic Nursing Practice, 5*, 67-76.

Courchene, V. S., Patelski, E., & Martin, J. (1991). A study of the health of pediatric nurses administering Cyclosporine A. *Pediatric Nursing, 17*, 497-500.

Cross, J. R. (1990). Betty Neuman. In J. B. George (Ed.), *Nursing theories: The base for professional nursing practice* (3rd ed.) (pp. 259-278). Norwalk, CT: Appleton & Lange.

Dale, M. L., & Savala, S. M. (1990). A new approach to the senior practicum. *Nursing Connections, 3*(1), 45-51.

DeBrun, K. T. (1988). *An investigation of the relationships among standing, sitting, recumbent postures, judgement of time duration and preferred personal space in adult females.* Unpublished doctoral dissertation, New York University.

Decker, S. D., & Young, E. (1991). Self-perceived needs of primary caregivers of home-hospice clients. *Journal of Community Health Nursing, 8*(3), 147-151.

DeLoughery, G. W., Gibbie, K. M., & Neuman, B. M. (1974). Teaching organizational concepts to nurses in community mental health. *Journal of Nursing Education, 13*, 18-24.

Delunas, L. R. (1990). Prevention of elder abuse: Betty Neuman health care systems approach. *Clinical Nurse Specialist, 4*, 54-58.

Derstine, J. B. (1992). Theory-based advanced rehabilitation nursing: Is it a reality? *Holistic Nursing Practice, 6*(2), 1-6.

Drew, L. L., Craig, D. M., & Beynon, C. E. (1989). The Neuman systems model for community health administration and practice: Provinces of Manitoba and Ontario, Canada. In B. Neuman (Ed.), *The Neuman systems model* (2nd ed.) (pp. 315-342). Norwalk, CT: Appleton & Lange.

Edwards, P. A., & Kittler, A. W. (1991). Integrating rehabilitation content in nursing curricula. *Rehabilitation Nursing, 16*(2), 70-73.

Field, P. A. (1987). The impact of nursing theory on the clinical decision making process. *Nurse Educator, 13*, 563-571.

Flannery, J. (1991). FAMILY-RESCUE: A family assessment tool for use by neuroscience nursing in the acute care setting. *Journal of Neuroscience Nursing, 23*, 111-115.

Flannery, J. C. (1988). Validity and reliability of levels of cognitive functioning assessment scale for adults with closed head injuries. *Dissertation Abstracts International, 48*, 3248B.

Foote, A. W., Piazza, D., & Schultz, M. (1990). The Neuman systems model: Application to a patient with a cervical spinal cord injury. *Journal of Neuroscience Nursing, 22*, 302-306.

Forchuk, C. (1991). Reconceptualizing the environment of the individual with a chronic mental illness. *Issues in Mental Health Nursing, 12*, 159-170.

Freiberger, D., Bryant, J., & Marino, B. (1992). The effects of different central venous line dressing changes on bacterial growth in a pediatric oncology population. *Journal of Pediatric Oncology Nursing, 9*(1), 2-7.

Fulbrook, P. R. (1991). The application of the Neuman systems model to intensive care. *Intensive Care Nursing, 7*(1), 28-39.

Gavan, C. A. S., Hastings-Tolsma, M. T., & Tryan, P. J. (1988). Explication of Neuman's model: A holistic systems approach to nutrition for health promotion in the life process. *Holistic Nursing Practice, 3*(1), 26-38.

Gavigan, M., Kline-O'Sullivan, C., & Klumpp-Lybrand, B. (1990). The effect of regular turning on CABG patients. *Critical Care Quarterly, 12*(4), 69-76.

Gibson, D. E. (1988). *A Q-analysis of interpersonal trust in the nurse-client relationship.* Unpublished doctoral dissertation, University of Alabama at Birmingham.

Gries, M., & Gernsler, J. (1988). Patient perceptions of the mechanical ventilation experience. *Focus on Critical Care, 15*, 52-59.

Harbin, P. D. O. (1989). *The Q-analysis of the stressors of adult female nursing students enrolled in baccalaureate schools of nursing.* Unpublished doctoral dissertation, University of Alabama at Birmingham.

Heffline, M. S. (1991). A comparative study of pharmacological versus nursing interventions in the treatment of postanesthesia shivering. *Journal of Post Anesthesia Nursing, 6*, 311-320.

Herrick, C. A., & Goodykoontz, L. (1989). Neuman's systems model for nursing practice as a conceptual framework for a family assessment. *Journal of Child and Adolescent Psychiatric Mental Health Nursing, 2*, 61-67.

Herrick, C. A., Goodykoontz, L., Herrick, R. H., & Kacket, B. (1991). Planning a continuum of care in child psychiatric nursing: A collaborative effort. *Journal of Child and Adolescent Psychiatric and Mental Health Nursing, 4*, 41-48.

Hiltz, D. (1990). The Neuman systems model: An analysis of a clinical situation. *Rehabilitation Nursing, 15,* 330-332.

Hinds, C. (1990). Personal and contextual factors predicting patients' reported quality of life: Exploring congruency with Betty Neuman's assumptions. *Journal of Advanced Nursing, 15,* 456-462.

Hinton-Walker, P., & Raborn, M. (1989). Application of the Neuman model in nursing administration and practice. In B. Henry, C. Arndt, M. DiVincenti, & A. Marriner-Tomey (Eds.), *Dimensions of nursing administration* (pp. 711-723). Boston: Blackwell Scientific Publications.

Hoch, C. C. (1987). Assessing delivery of nursing care . . . Roy adaptation model and the Neuman health care systems model . . . increasing life satisfaction in retired individuals. *Journal of Gerontological Nursing, 13*(1), 10-17.

Hoeman, S. P., & Winters, D. M. (1990). Theory-based case management: High cervical spinal cord injury. *Home Healthcare Nurse, 8*(1), 25-33.

Huch, M. H. (1991). Perspectives on health. *Nursing Science Quarterly, 1*(1), 33-40.

Johnson, S. E. (1989). A picture is worth a thousand words: Helping students visualize a conceptual model. *Nurse Educator, 14*(3), 21-24.

Kaku, R. V. (1992). Severity of low back pain: A comparison between participants who did and did not receive counseling. *AAOHN-Journal, 10*(2), 81-89.

Knight, J. B. (1990). The Betty Neuman systems model applied to practice: A client with multiple sclerosis. *Journal of Advanced Nursing, 15,* 447-455.

Laschinger, H. K., & Duff, V. (1991). Attitudes of practicing nurses towards theory-based nursing practice. *Canadian Journal of Nursing Administration, 1*(1), 6-10.

Leja, A. M. (1989). Using guided imagery to combat postsurgical depression. *Journal of Gerontological Nursing, 15*(4), 6-11.

Lindell, M., & Olsson, H. (1991). Can combined oral contraceptives be made more effective by means of a nursing care model? *Journal of Advanced Nursing, 16,* 475-479.

Loescher, L. J., Clark, L., Atwood, J. R., Leigh, S., & Lamb, G. (1990). The impact of the cancer experience on long-term survivors. *Oncology Nursing Forum, 17,* 223-229.

Louis, M. (1989). An intervention to reduce anxiety levels for nurses working with long-term care clients using Neuman's model. In J. P. Riehl-Sisca (Ed.), *Conceptual models for nursing practice* (3rd ed.) (pp. 95-103). Norwalk, CT: Appleton & Lange.

Lowry, L. W. (1988). Operationalizing the Neuman systems model: A course in concepts and process. *Nurse Educator, 13*(3), 19-22.

Lowry, L. W., & Jopp, M. C. (1989). An evaluation instrument for assessing an associate degree nursing curriculum based on the Neuman systems model. In J. P. Riehl-Sisca (Ed.), *Conceptual models for nursing practice* (3rd ed.) (pp. 73-85). Norwalk, CT: Appleton & Lange.

Maynihan, M. M. (1990). Nursing theories in practice: Implementation of the Neuman systems model in an acute care nursing department. *NLN Publication, #15-2350,* 263-273.

McDaniel, G. M. S. (1989). *The effects of two methods of dangling on heart rate and blood pressure in post-operative abdominal hysterectomy patients.* Unpublished doctoral dissertation, University of Alabama at Birmingham.

Mirenda, R. (1986). The Neuman model in practice. *Senior Nurse, 5*(3), 26-27.

Mirenda, R. (1986). Neuman systems model. In P. Winstead-Fry (Ed.), *Case studies in nursing theory. NLN Publication, #15-2152,* 127-166.

Mischke-Berkey, K., Warner, P., & Hanson, S. (1989). Family health assessment and intervention. In P. J. Bomar (Ed.), *Nurses and family health promotion: Concepts, assessment and interventions* (pp. 115-154). Baltimore, MD: Williams and Wilkins.

Moore, S. L., & Munro, M. F. (1990). The Neuman systems model applied to mental health nursing of older adults. *Journal of Advanced Nursing, 15,* 293-299.

Moynihan, M. M. (1990). Implementation of the Neuman systems model in an acute care nursing department. In M. E. Parker (Ed.), *Nursing theories in practice* (pp. 263-273). New York: National League for Nursing.

Mrkonich, D. E., Hessian, M., & Miller, M. W. (1989). A cooperative process in curriculum development using the Neuman health-care systems model. In J. P. Riehl-Sisca (Ed.), *Conceptual models for nursing practice* (3rd ed.) (pp. 87-94). Norwalk, CT: Appleton & Lange.

Neuman, B. (1982). *The Neuman systems model: Application to nursing education and practice.* New York: Appleton-Century-Crofts.

Neuman, B. (1989). The Neuman nursing process format: Family. In J. P. Riehl-Sisca (Ed.), *Conceptual models for nursing practice* (3rd ed.) (pp. 49-62). Norwalk, CT: Appleton & Lange.

Neuman, B. (1989). *The Neuman systems model* (2nd ed.). Norwalk, CT: Appleton & Lange.

Neuman, B. (1990). The Neuman systems model: A theory for practice. In M. E. Parker (Ed.), *Nursing theories in practice* (pp. 241-261). New York: National League for Nursing.

Neuman, B., & Wyatt, M. (1981, January 20). Prospects for change: Some evaluation reflections from one articulated baccalaureate program. *Journal of Nursing Education,* 40-46.

Neuman, B., & Young, J. (1972). A model for teaching total person approach to patient problems. *Nursing Research, 21,* 264-269.

Neuman, B. M. (1990). Health as a continuum based on the Neuman systems model. *Nursing Science Quarterly, 3,* 129-135.

Norman, S. E. (1991). The relationship between hardiness and sleep disturbances in HIV-infected men. *Dissertation Abstracts International, 51,* 4780B.

Norris, E. W. (1989). *Physiologic response to exercise in clients with mitral valve prolapse syndrome.* Unpublished doctoral dissertation, University of Alabama at Birmingham.

Parker, M. E. (Ed.). (1991). *Nursing theories in practice.* New York: National League for Nursing.

Peoples, L. T. (1991). *The relationship between selected client, provider, and agency variables and the utilization of home care services.* Unpublished doctoral dissertation, University of Alabama at Birmingham.

Piazza, D., Foote, A., Wright, P., & Holcombe, J. (1992). Neuman systems model used as a guide for the nursing care of an 8-year-old child with leukemia. *Journal of Pediatric Nursing, 9*(1), 17-24.

Pierce, J. D., & Hutton, E. (1992). Applying the new concepts of the Neuman systems model. *Nursing Forum, 27*(1), 15-18.

Quayhagen, M. P., & Roth, P. A. (1989). From models to measures in assessment of mature families. *Journal of Professional Nursing, 5,* 144-151.

Reed, K. (1993). Adapting the Neuman systems model for family nursing. *Nursing Science Quarterly, 6*(2), 93-97.

Reed, K. S. (1989). Family theory related to the Neuman systems model. In B. Neuman (Ed.), *The Neuman systems model* (2nd ed.) (pp. 385-395). Norwalk, CT: Appleton & Lange.

Riehl-Sisca, J. P. (1989). *Conceptual models for nursing practice* (3rd ed.). Norwalk, CT: Appleton & Lange.

Ross, M. M., Bourbonnais, F. F., & Carroll, G. (1987). Curricular design and the Betty Neuman systems model: A new approach to learning. *International Nursing Review, 34*(3/273), 75-79.

Ross, M. M., & Helmer, H. (1988). A comparative analysis of Neuman's model using the individual and family as the units of care. *Public Health Nursing, 5,* 30-36.

Rowe, M. L. (1989). *The relationship of commitment and social support to the life satisfaction of caregivers to patients with Alzheimer's disease.* Unpublished doctoral dissertation, University of Texas at Austin.

Schlosser, S. P. (1986). The effect of anticipatory guidance on mood state in primparas experiencing unplanned cesarean delivery (metropolitan area, Southeast). *Dissertation Abstracts International, 46,* 2627B.

Simmons, L., & Borgdon, C. (1991). The clinical nurse specialist in HIV care. *Kansas Nurse, 66*(1), 6-7.

Sipple, J. E. A. (1989). *A model for curriculum change based on retrospective analysis.* Unpublished doctoral dissertation, University of South Carolina, Columbia.

Sirles, A. T., Brown, K., & Hilver, J. C. (1991). Effects of back school education and exercise in back injured municipal workers. *AAOHN Journal, 39*(1), 7-12.

Smith, M. C. (1989). Neuman's model in practice. *Nursing Science Quarterly, 2,* 24-25.

Speck, B. J. (1990). The effect of guided imagery upon first semester nursing students performing their first injections. *Journal of Nursing Education, 29,* 346-350.

Story, E. L., & DuGas, B. W. (1988). A teaching strategy to facilitate conceptual model implementation in practice. *Journal of Continuing Education in Nursing, 19,* 244-247.

Story, E. L., & Ross, M. M. (1986). Family centered community health nursing and the Betty Neuman systems model. *Nursing Papers, Perspectives in Nursing, 18,* 77-88.

Terhaar, M. F. (1989). The influence of physiologic stability, behavioral stability and family stability on the preterm infant's length of stay in the neonatal intensive care unit. *Dissertation Abstracts International, 50,* 1328B.

Torkington, S. (1988). Nourishing the infant. *Senior Nurse, 8*(2), 24-25.

Vaughn, M., Cheatwood, S., Sirles, A. T., & Brown, K. C. (1989). The effect of progressive muscle relaxation on stress among clerical workers. *American Association of Occupational Health Nurses Journal, 37,* 302-306.

Vincent, J. L. M. (1988). A Q analysis of the stressors of fathers with an infant in an intensive care unit. *Dissertation Abstracts International, 49,* 3111B.

Wallingford, P. (1989). The neurologically impaired and dying child: Applying the Neuman systems model. *Issues in Comprehensive Pediatric Nursing, 12,* 139-157.

Webb, C. A. (1988). *Q cross-sectional study of hope, physical status, cognitions and meaning and purpose of pre- and post-retirement adults.* Unpublished doctoral dissertation, University of Pittsburgh.

Weinberger, S. L. (1991). Analysis of clinical situation using the Neuman systems model. *Rehabilitation Nursing, 16,* 278, 280-281.

Whatley, J. H. (1988). *Effects of health locus of control and social network on risk-taking in adolescents.* Unpublished doctoral dissertation, University of Alabama at Birmingham.

Wheeler, K. (1989). Self-psychology's contributions to understanding stress and implications for nursing. *Journal of Advanced Medical Surgical Nursing, 1*(4), 1-10.

Wiens, A. G. (1985). Rehabilitation assessment—A nursing perspective . . . the Neuman nursing model. *Rehabilitation Nursing, 10*(2), 25-27.

Williamson, J. W. (1989). *The influence of self-selected monotonous sounds on the night sleep pattern of postoperative open heart surgery patients.* Unpublished doctoral dissertation, University of Alabama at Birmingham.

About the Author

Karen S. Reed is an Associate Professor in the College of Nursing at the University of Akron, Ohio. Her association with Dr. Neuman began in 1979 at Ohio University, where Dr. Neuman first encouraged her to explore the idea of family as a client system. That work was published in the 1982 edition of *The Neuman systems model.* She has spent the past 12 years continuing to incorporate family constructs within the Neuman model, and was a contributor to the 1989 edition of the Neuman book. In addition, she has presented the family-focused material at several national and international conferences on nursing theory and family nursing. Her most recent work has focused on developing a family assessment model based on the Neuman systems model (NFAM). Her current research interests focus on testing the family assessment model and the impact of perinatal loss on families. Recent publications include an article on miscarriages in *Image,* an article on the development of NFAM in *Nursing Science Quarterly,* and two book chapters on family and psychiatric disorders in children in the pediatric textbook *Child Health Nursing.*